YOUR CAREER AS A
PODIATRIST
Doctor of Podiatric Medicine (DPM)

HEALTHCARE FOR THE FOOT

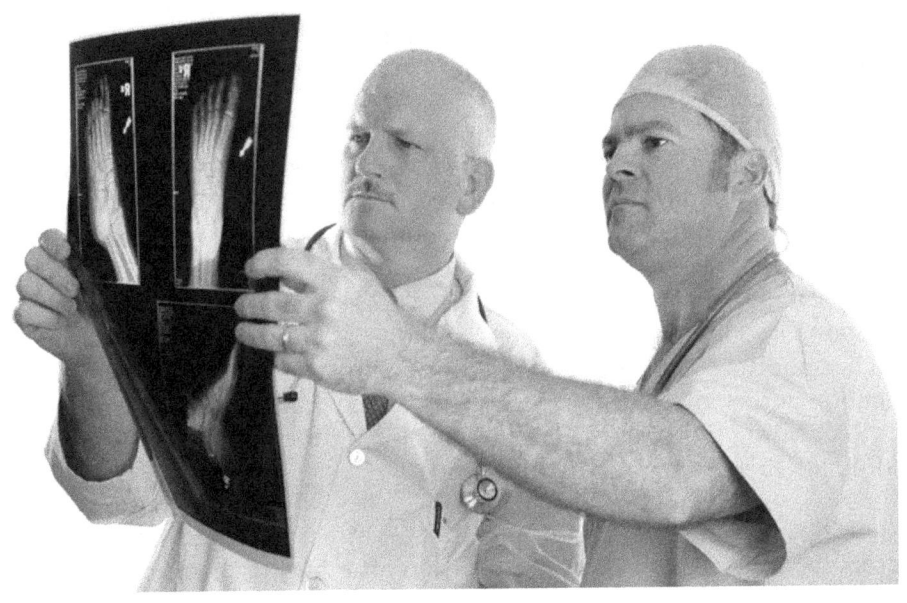

THE GREAT RENAISSANCE ARTIST Leonardo da Vinci said, "The human foot is a masterpiece of engineering and a work of art." It is hard to disagree with that. The human foot can be a thing of beauty, and usually functions extremely well. But when anything goes wrong with it, the human foot can be a source of nearly unbearable pain and frustration.

Considering the amount of work it has to do, bearing up under great pressure as we walk or run, or even when we are only standing still, it is truly remarkable what the fragile human foot can manage. There are 26 bones in the human foot and ankle. That is one out of every four of the bones in the whole human body! In addition, there are 33 joints and 100 muscles, tendons and ligaments. No wonder the foot requires its own special doctor. That specialist is the podiatrist.

Podiatrists diagnose and treat illnesses, injuries, and deformities of the human feet and ankles including the foot muscles, joints, or bones. They work with children and seniors, athletes and the obese, civilians and veterans. The problems that podiatrists deal with can be relatively simple, like a corn that needs removing. They can also be extremely complicated, even to the point of requiring surgery. From the simplest to the most complicated cases, the podiatrist is rarely dealing with a patient who is not in significant pain.

The term chiropodist is often confused with podiatrist. It is an older term for what was once the same profession. In the US, only the term podiatrist is used in reference to the fully-trained professional foot specialist. About 50 years ago, the US training schools changed their names to only include the word podiatry. Graduates were thereafter awarded a Doctor of Podiatric Medicine (DPM) degree.

In the United Kingdom, in fact, there is no difference between the terms chiropodist and podiatrist. They are used interchangeably. In Canada and other countries, podiatrists are also sometimes referred to as chiropodists. But the Canadian Podiatric Medical Association (CPME) explains that while there are many similarities between the two, there are "differences in the educational requirements as well as the scope of practice for podiatrists and chiropodists." The CPME notes that podiatrists have a more extensive education and enjoy a broader scope of practice than what chiropodists are able to perform. Chiropodists are not entitled to practice at all in British Columbia, Alberta, Manitoba and Quebec.

One of the more interesting notes about podiatry is that many of these doctors say they decided on this profession after having themselves been treated for a foot or ankle injury. The injuries were often sports related and many podiatrists are athletes. Their own personal experience of being treated by a podiatrist was the key, which suggests there are many great podiatrists out there.

Some podiatrists are clear that they chose this field because they were impatient to get to work. Getting licensed as a podiatrist requires a shorter period of education and training than some other medical fields.

Podiatrists are more in demand than ever. Podiatry is projected to be one of the fastest growing healthcare occupations over the next decade, increasing at a rate double that for all occupations. The increase reflects a demand born largely out of the growing needs of two demographic groups. The US has an aging population that will face increased health challenges that are difficult to avoid, as many are part of the natural aging process.

In addition, obesity is on the increase as is diabetes and both of these conditions can be the source of foot and ankle injuries and illnesses. Even the growing number of people today who are actively seeking to stay healthy through vigorous exercise contributes to the need for podiatrists, specifically those podiatrists who specialize in sports medicine.

Podiatrists are in demand and the demand is growing, and so is the educational and training system.

The profession, its individual members and organizations, are all working toward expanding the already rapid rate of growth. Changes are being made that will create more paths to professional acceptance than have previously been available, and the next few years and beyond should be ones of increasing opportunities for students who wish to become podiatrists.

THINGS TO DO NOW

BECOMING A PODIATRIST IS A LONG and challenging process. There are several things you can do while still in high school in order to prepare for this. The first, obviously, is to take all the science classes that are available at your school, especially biology. It is also worthwhile to go beyond the classroom and join a biology club where you can delve deeper into the workings of the human body, especially the feet and ankles.

Many podiatrists were athletes in school. If you are on a high school team, you can get to know whoever is responsible for the team's health and well-being. Pay special attention to what they do, especially for injuries of the feet and legs. If you are not on a team, volunteer to help the trainer or nurse responsible for team healthcare.

Take communications classes as well, in order to begin developing the writing and speaking skills that will be a necessary part of your work as a podiatrist. You might even consider joining the debate team, not so much for developing your speaking skills, but more importantly to begin to develop good listening skills that will be critical when determining the full scope of each patient's problems.

You can try to find opportunities to volunteer or even find part- time or after schoolwork in facilities that provide some type of healthcare. Spending time in these types of places will help you to become accustomed to being around people who are ill and injured. You may also want to seek out podiatrists in your area looking for ones who will let you shadow them as they see their patients. The American Podiatric Medical Association (APMA) might be able to help you find someone in your area who would be agreeable to the idea.

Of course, podiatrists may not let you observe everything they do, but you should be able to discover details that would not otherwise be available unless you were a patient yourself, or until you began making rounds while in your second year in podiatry school. Shadowing a working podiatrist will give you the clearest idea of whether you have made a good choice for your future.

This is also a great time to begin reading the professional journals of podiatry. Much of it may be beyond your scope at first but you might discover that the articles become clearer as you continue reading. Even if the medical terms are hard to track down, it will give you an idea of the important issues for the profession, the developments taking place in equipment and techniques, and the questions that podiatrists are asking each other about their work.

Get to know your own feet and your own ankles. If your career is going to be all about other people's feet, having a strong sense of your own – where they hurt; if you walk on your heels, your toes, or on the outside of your feet; or if they turn one way or the other, for example. Get your family members to volunteer their feet and ankles for inspection, as well. That way, you can begin getting used to handling other people's feet. It's a great way to begin!

HISTORY OF PODIATRY AS A CAREER

ANKHMAHOR WAS "GRAND VIZIER, First under the King, Overseer of the Great House" of the pharaoh Teti who reigned over Egypt around 2300 BC. Ankhmahor's tomb, which was first excavated toward the end of the 19th century, is known as the "Tomb of the Physician." This is not because Ankhmahor himself was a doctor but because of the carvings on the entrance to his tomb that depict people having the calluses on their feet scrapped by what archaeologists believe to be professional foot care providers, the first known podiatrists. Many Egyptologists believe podiatry was already being practiced even earlier than this period, and may very well have been a standard treatment throughout the several thousand years of ancient Egyptian civilization.

The Greek physician Hippocrates, credited as the Father of Western Medicine and author of the Hippocratic Oath still followed by physicians to this day, wrote extensively about foot care and is also credited with creating a scalpel to be used specifically for scraping away calluses and corns.

Podiatry continued to be practiced throughout the following centuries, mostly by workers known as "corn cutters." Any other treatment of the feet and ankles was left to practitioners of general medicine, who history records as believing corn cutting was beneath their professional skills. Although much in demand, corn cutting was not for most of history a lucrative profession, and corn cutters traveled around from town to town to offer their services and their homemade salves and other medications. By the late 17th century, however, some corn cutters were seeing substantial success if they could provide their services to the nobility.

In the late 18th century, information about the proper care and treatment of foot injuries and illnesses was organized into a published text for the first time since Hippocrates, entitled *L'Art de Soigner les Pieds* by a Frenchman, Nicholas-Laurent LaForest. Corn cutters began to settle in offices where they sometimes served as dentists, as well. According to British business records, the city of London had its first registered podiatrist in 1800 (referred to as a chiropodist in those days). The first English volume on foot care was produced two years later. By 1840, there were three registered podiatrists in London, in 1845 the first medical text on foot care appeared, and by 1880 there were 40 practitioners.

In 1895, the first association for foot specialists was formed in the United States and named the Pedic Society of New York. Within 20 years the first school dedicated to training foot specialists, was opened in the US, and training programs and schools began to appear in Europe, as well.

The National Association of Chiropodists was established in 1912 with 225 chiropodist members. This was the organization that evolved into the present-day American Podiatric Medical Association (APMA). The profession went through a period of reform in the 1960s, led by APMA. The efforts were primarily focused on upgrading the educational structure supporting the profession, but these efforts also resulted in a better informational system for professionals to communicate with each other, and for the profession to communicate with their patients and the public.

Today, the APMA and its affiliate, the Council on Podiatric Medical Education (CPME), are engaged in ongoing campaigns to promote recognition of the profession and to improve the quality of the accredited colleges of podiatric medicine.

WHERE YOU WILL WORK

PODIATRISTS PRACTICE IN A VARIETY OF settings, including:

- Private practices
- Children's hospitals
- General hospitals
- Veterans hospitals
- Orthopedic and sports medicine clinics
- Rehabilitation clinics
- Nursing homes
- Managed care organizations

Private practices can refer to a single podiatrist working alone, or it can be a group practice with several podiatrists sharing support staff, rent, and other expenses. Podiatrists work in the military as well as in civilian society. Some are attached to private business to treat employees, especially if it is the type of business that creates stress for the feet and ankles, as can be the case in manufacturing, retail, and a variety of service industries.

Podiatrists also teach, usually in the podiatric medical schools. They can also teach by offering presentations about preventive care in schools, community organizations, and private businesses. Podiatrists also do research in university and hospital laboratories, and they can also work for medical supply companies, representing the companies' products to other podiatrists.

Podiatrists will work closely with other physicians and surgeons. Some podiatrists, but not all, are themselves surgeons. They also work with registered nurses, and medical assistants and, especially in private practice, with administrative and clerical support staff.

For podiatrists who perform surgery and who also teach, there will be workdays that will take them from one location to another throughout the day. They might start the day with a faculty meeting; then move on to the classroom for a lesson; then to their clinical rounds, accompanied by students; and finally to surgery in an operating room. It is even possible that they will go on to see patients in a private clinic before the day is through.

For the most part, however, podiatrists tend to spend their day in a clinical setting, seeing one patient after another, usually during regular business hours. There are also podiatrists who work for outsourcing organizations that send them on the road to clinics, nursing homes, and other facilities, where there is no podiatrist on staff. The traveling podiatrist can cover a territory that encompasses several healthcare facilities, making scheduled rounds and being available for emergencies.

A similar role, but one with a larger scope, is that of podiatrists who participate in global health projects through a university, government, or non-governmental organization. Illnesses and injuries of the feet and ankles happen everywhere and in emerging nations there are typically not enough doctors, especially not podiatrists, to treat everyone in need. Participating in such a project may be a one-time event or something that occurs infrequently. There are others who have made such work the focus of their careers, just as medical professionals in other disciplines have done.

THE WORK YOU WILL DO

PODIATRISTS ARE DOCTORS WHO SPECIALIZE in the medical and surgical care of people with foot, ankle, and lower leg problems. They both diagnose and treat illnesses and injuries, and can perform surgery involving the lower extremities.

Specific tasks that a podiatrist could perform in order to assess the overall condition of a patient's feet, ankles, or lower legs might typically include:

- Allowing patients to describe their concerns
- Reviewing the patient's medical history
- Performing a physical examination of the patient, which may include the use of X-rays and other laboratory tests such as urinalysis and blood tests.

From the assessment, the podiatrist will next diagnose foot, ankle, and lower leg problems and then advise the patient on the possible treatments that would apply to the condition. With the patient's agreement, the podiatrist moves to provide treatment for the ailments, which could involve anything from prescribing medications or shoe inserts (orthotics), to scraping calluses and removing corns, to performing surgery, which can include repairing breaks and fractures, removing bone spurs, and correcting deformities and other physical problems.

Once the podiatrist has provided treatment to the patient, further advice and instructions will be offered to the patient on the proper care and general wellness techniques to follow. Podiatrists may also coordinate patient care with other physicians or refer patients to other specialists if they perceive a need for additional medical attention.

Some of the specific tasks the podiatrist might perform include:

- Biomechanical assessments
- Dermatological assessments
- Diabetic foot care
- Foot care advice and evaluation
- Kinesiology taping

- Nail care
- Nail surgery with use of local anesthetic
- Orthotic prescription and casting
- Podiatric acupuncture
- Screening for type 2 diabetes (neurological & vascular)
- Sports injury assessment, management and prevention
- Ulcer management and treatment
- Verruca therapy

The work of a podiatrist can be broken down into six specialty areas. Podiatrists spend at least three years in a residency program after earning their degrees, during which time they choose which of the six areas will be their specialty. It is worth noting that some choose more than one, which does enhance the chances for finding a position in a clinic or private practice when the residency is completed.

The areas of specialization within the field of podiatric medicine include:

Podiatric Orthopedics

This area focuses on treatment through the use of special footwear, orthotic and prosthetic devices of foot and leg structures and functions that are damaged in one way or another. Physical therapy is another form of treatment within this area of focus.

Podiatric Primary Care

Podiatrists focus on primary care in terms of prevention, diagnosis, and treatment of foot and ankle conditions, as they exist in the overall healthcare environment of patients and their families.

Podiatric Sports Medicine

This area focuses on the disorders of the feet and ankles which have been caused or aggravated by pursuing an athletic activity. Sports podiatrists seek to prevent problems through education, but must also diagnose and treat those disorders when they do occur.

Podiatric Surgery

Podiatric surgeons use a variety of operative techniques and procedures in order to repair damages that have occurred to the feet and ankles.

Podopediatrics

Primary care – prevention, diagnosis, and treatment – with a focus on the foot, ankle, and leg problems faced by children.

Wound Care and Management

Podiatrists focusing on this specialty deal with the prevention of wounds, ulcers, and injuries of the lower extremities, especially related to diabetes and other chronic systemic diseases; and the care and treatment of these problems when they do occur.

Most podiatrists work full time. It is not unusual for their offices to be open in the evenings and on weekends to accommodate the work schedules of patients. Podiatrists working in hospitals may occasionally be called on to staff night or weekend shifts. They may also be on call even when they are not on duty.

Podiatrists can be research scientists as well as practitioners. Research is usually conducted in a university, especially institutions with their own clinics, but can also happen in the facilities of medical equipment manufacturers. Part of the work of research podiatrists is to share their findings in peer-reviewed publications and also by presenting their findings at professional gatherings.

Podiatrists can also be teachers. It is typical for teachers in the podiatric medical schools to be practicing physicians, and sometimes even surgeons, as well as working in the classroom. Podiatrists engaged at universities may work exclusively for the university in its classrooms, labs, and clinics. Others may split their time between the university and private practice.

Whatever their role in academia, part time or full time, the podiatrist's job will include preparing lessons, and marking exams and papers, and determining final grades. It is also likely that students will ask for letters of recommendation.

Similarly, whether a podiatrist is working in a hospital, a clinic, or in private practice, it will be necessary to maintain patient records and submit insurance information. Even if there is a strong administrative support staff, the doctor is still going to participate to some degree in the paperwork process.

In any specialty or type of work, part of the podiatrist's job is to stay abreast of developments in their field. To a large extent this is done through following the professional journals for podiatrists. It can also include traveling to attend professional conferences and other gatherings in order to hear peer delivered research papers.

Some podiatrists work in sales. There are many podiatry equipment and supplies manufacturers, as well as companies that sell multiple podiatry supply brands. While most rely on persons with business backgrounds or sales experience in the medical field, there is always interest in employing representatives who have first-hand knowledge of how the supplies are used.

Looking ahead at what the work of the podiatrist will be in the near future, there is a good chance that there may be more severe cases on three fronts. First, there is the overall aging of the population, which will bring in more seniors than ever with the specific lower limb ailments related to the aging process. Podiatrists remind us that with the amount of stress we put on our feet in a lifetime, foot problems are very hard to avoid. Besides the wear and tear of the passing years, problems related to drying skin and other skin conditions increase with age, as do issues of swelling, circulation, and bones becoming more fragile. Podiatrists treat all these as well as other age-related developments, such as arthritic ankles.

There is also expected to be an increase in the numbers of illnesses and injuries related to obesity and the health problems that are related to being significantly overweight, especially diabetes, but also cardiovascular diseases and cancer. According to the Centers for Disease Control and Prevention over 78 million adults and 12.5 million children in the US are obese. That translates to about 36 percent of all adults and 17 percent of all children.

According to the Institute for Preventive Foot Health (IPFH), obese people face increased forefoot pain and increased frequency or probability of both specific foot conditions and nonspecific foot pain, as well as chronic plantar heel pain, tendinitis, gout, and osteoarthritis. The IPFH also cites research indicating that the feet of obese children are often in such discomfort that the children increasingly refrain from physical activity.

Obesity increases the risk of type 2 diabetes. In fact, nearly nine out of 10 people living with this condition are overweight or obese. This is the result of the added pressure on their body's ability to use naturally occurring insulin to control blood sugar levels. Nerve disorders result from that situation and these are linked directly to several extreme conditions for the feet and legs of the diabetes sufferer. These nerve disorders can result in the need to amputate feet, toes, and legs.

The profession also may see an increase in patients who are athletes and who participate in sports and fitness routines. Large segments of the population, young and old alike are dedicated to maintaining their health. Exercise plays a big part in that effort and unfortunately injuries to the feet, legs, and ankles are a frequent occurrence. The range of injuries can be extensive, from mild sprains to broken bones. It is worth remembering that even mild problems of the feet and legs can be painful.

One other group that may have an increased need for podiatrists is combat veterans. The state of world affairs is extremely unsettled and it is hard to know whether the US military will be more engaged in the coming years. Recent years have shown that injuries to the feet, legs, and ankles happen often to those in active military service. Podiatrists have a big role to play in dealing with the problems of veterans.

PODIATRISTS TALK ABOUT THEIR CAREERS

I Became a Podiatrist Because as a Child I Wanted to be Taller

"I started playing organized football when I was about 10 or 11 but I was small for my age. I began reading books about the body and almost immediately I knew I wanted to be a doctor. I didn't decide on podiatry until I was in my junior year as an undergraduate. I was thinking about becoming an orthopedist but my adviser suggested I think about becoming a podiatrist. There was a shadowing program available at one of the podiatric colleges and I was accepted into it. So I got to follow a podiatrist around for a week, sitting in on patient visits, making rounds in a hospital, and observing in a surgery. I was hooked. Also, I have to admit, I liked the idea that the three-year residency for podiatry was half the six year residency needed to become an orthopedic medical doctor.

After I completed my residency and passed my board certification exam I was invited to join a very successful surgical practice. I made very good money but I wasn't satisfied. I was helping people but it felt like an assembly line. It wasn't personal enough. I had liked academia and doing research so when I saw a position open up at one of the colleges I jumped at it.

like what I'm doing now. I teach, oversee curriculum, do research, do rounds in the clinic the school operates, and also perform surgery at the clinic. My students come with me on the rounds as part of their training.

I go out of my way to talk to my patients, educate them, rather than trying to simplify everything and talking down to them. Even so, there are patients who expect miracles no matter what you tell them. The only other complaint I have is about the whole business structure. Some doctors choose more expensive options, like the type of splint they use, because it may be a bit more comfortable for the patient. That's okay, except the differences can be extreme. It drives up costs, insurance companies turn down the charge, and sometimes the hospital winds up paying for it. The system is really messed up.

I don't make as much money as I did in private practice but I'm so much happier. I'm very pleased with what I do and being able to help people. That's what it's all about or should be all about."

Podiatry Combined All the Things in Medicine I Was Looking For

"The costs of going to podiatry school were lower than those of other medical schools, which I liked because I didn't want to be deep in debt when I graduated. I saw that a lot of medical students in other fields made choices about where they were going to live and work because of the huge debt they carried out of school. I wanted to make a choice that was based on what I wanted, not because I was being forced to do it. I am very passionate about medicine, I think it is perhaps the most rewarding work that you can do on earth, but it is still a job like any other. I wanted to work to live, not the other way around. It is very simple, a career in podiatry allows for that level of balance.

My specialist skills focus on treating hard skin, infections, ailments, and defects and injuries of the foot and lower leg. I prescribe custom made orthotics and other aids and appliances, along with dry needling and laser treatment for verrucae. I also use cryotherapy.

So many of my patients have foot and nail conditions that are the result of major health disorders, meaning, usually, diabetes. These are known as the high-risk patients, along with elderly patients. This is serious business. A lot of these people have an increased risk of amputation. More often, what I do is nail and soft tissue surgery that only requires local anesthesia. I offer my patients advice on improving mobility, independence, and the quality of their lives. I teach them skills for preventative care.

I also work closely with other medical practitioners such as doctors, nurses, health visitors, physiotherapists, and other healthcare professionals. That's one of the best parts of the job, working with a multidisciplinary team. I do that most often when it comes to sports-related injuries to legs and feet. The sports injuries are interesting because the tools, things like kinetic strappings, dressings, insole materials, and video gait-analysis equipment are different from what I need for the other types of therapy.

Lately I've been studying other languages because my patient base has been getting more diverse. I usually have an interpreter available if the patient doesn't speak English or only speaks it a little. But I want to know more and be able to explain some things myself."

I Was in the Navy, a General Practitioner, and a Member of a Triathlon Team

"I became interested in sports injuries affecting the foot, ankle and lower limbs and I went back to school to study podiatry. Going back to school set the stage for continuing my education to this day. I enjoy learning new things and tracking the most current developments in podiatry. A lot is happening! There are new products being developed all the time and you have to stay on your toes to be able to tell the ones with value from the ones that are simply a waste of your time and your patients' money.

The clinic where I'm now a partner provides a comprehensive podiatry service, including sports injury assessment, exercise rehabilitation, nail surgery, routine foot care, and a foot and lower leg screening service for the diabetic patient. We specialize in custom-made prescription orthotics using our 3D foot scanning system, one of the things I read about and got really interested in as a result of my research. We have a pretty heavy case load at the clinic so tools that save time and energy are really important to us.

Maybe it's the Navy in my background but I am very concerned to make sure we follow all the guidelines and procedures relating to health and safety that the profession advises. I think it is critical to do that for the patients and for the staff, too. Following the rules doesn't mean I'm not passionate about being a podiatrist, because I am very passionate about it. It is a great career. So many of the problems I deal with are the same, and yet every patient is different and unique in some way. I'm always involved."

I Treat a Wide Range of Musculoskeletal Disorders of the Lower Limb Arising From Foot Function

"A primary focus of my practice is on the function of the foot during the gait cycle. I have a specialist interest in the developing foot of children, but I provide care to patients of all ages. I am also a consulting podiatrist at several hospitals, including a children's hospital, providing advice to colleagues on any and all problems that can affect the foot and ankle. I have my own clinic, too, which I established almost 25 years ago.

I'm very proud of the number of people I've been able to help over the years, including doctors I've advised as well as patients. My work has included teaching surgery and I serve on several committees of the Podiatrists Association. Much of my work is centered around encouraging podiatrists to continue their education even though they are out in the world practicing their profession.

I'm also very happy that I chose a profession that has allowed me to have a family life and still make a good income. I've been able to see my kids grow up and I could afford to send them to college. A lot of doctors make more money but they miss the family part of life. It's not that I didn't work hard, but somehow podiatry allowed me to establish boundaries."

I Knew I Wanted to Be a Doctor Even Before I Got to High School

"It wasn't until I went to a podiatrist for my own foot problem that I knew podiatry was what I wanted to do. I had a lot of neighbors who were doctors, dentists, and healthcare professionals like physical therapists. Because they knew me and my family they let me visit them at work and shadow them, as they liked to say.

Toward the end of high school I had my first encounter with a podiatrist, not one of neighbors but someone I had to see because I had developed a large plantar wart on my heel and couldn't walk without it hurting like crazy! I was used to observing how doctors behaved and I was very impressed by the podiatrist's manner. So many of the other doctors I had spent time with came across as intimidating but this doctor wasn't. He gave me and my parents a diagnosis very quickly, his treatment was straightforward, and he was really great when it came to telling me how to prevent further foot problems from occurring. That was it. I forgot about being a dentist or a general practitioner or any of the other professions I'd observed.

As soon as I started college everything was aimed at becoming a podiatrist. I went to Chile for two years of volunteer service for my church. While there I learned the Spanish language and adapted to a new culture. I also discovered that I have a talent for communicating and relating with others. I was able to discuss with the people I met ways of improving their lifestyle in a positive and effective way.

Even before I got to podiatry school I had observed a variety of foot and ankle problems and was already learning how to treat them. There were fungal problems, infected toes, and wart treatments. Podiatrists I shadowed didn't let me observe surgeries but I did get to sit in on surgical follow-ups. Even better than learning about the treatments was seeing how the doctors interacted with their patients. They made the patients feel relaxed and answered questions about their treatment. That might have been the most important thing I got from the experience, realizing how important it is to let your patients know that you care, that you are there for them.

I try to share that with students and new podiatrists whenever I have a chance to interact with them. I strongly urge anyone who is considering becoming a podiatrist, or any kind of doctor to do what I did. Get out there and see for yourself. Books are great but nothing beats seeing things for yourself!"

PERSONAL QUALIFICATIONS

LIKE ALL DOCTORS, PODIATRISTS need to be compassionate people. The patients a podiatrist sees are almost certain to be in pain. Some will be in mild pain and some in extreme pain. Podiatrists need to combine that compassion with the ability to think scientifically and critically about the conditions in which they find their patients. They must be able to apply their education and training in an analytical fashion in order to correctly diagnose a patient and determine the best course of treatment.

Hand-in-hand with this ability to think critically is the ability to be detail oriented. Illnesses and injuries may have some obvious elements to them, but each is unique to a particular individual and must be examined closely to make sure that no aspect is overlooked in developing a diagnosis.

The compassion that the podiatrist may feel and the details of the diagnosis both need to be communicated to the patient. The podiatrist cannot afford to hide or minimize any critical information. Communications skills, spoken as well as written, are extremely important in the work of the podiatrist at every stage of interaction with the patient, from the first meeting, through the assessment and diagnosis, the treatment, and, very importantly, the follow-up.

Communications skills also refer to the ability to listen well. Podiatrists must pay attention to their patients, listening for those remarks that may clarify understanding of the patient's condition, alerting the podiatrist to some small detail that might otherwise have been overlooked. The podiatrist must be able to make patients feel comfortable and secure so that they will open up and share that kind of detail that, if they do not feel safe, might go unspoken.

Another important quality for the podiatrist is good manual dexterity. This is, of course, especially important for those podiatrists who perform surgery. It is even important for podiatrists who do not perform surgery, because of their need to be hands-on with the feet and ankles of their patients. Having good manual dexterity is also necessary when using the diagnostic and surgical implements that the podiatrist will employ in the performance of their professional duties.

ATTRACTIVE FEATURES

YOU CANNOT UNDERESTIMATE THE PERSONAL and emotional satisfaction that comes from helping people. The ability to relieve pain is a gift and podiatrists are very pleased at being able to do that. Many also add that their work tends to produce very tangible results fairly quickly, and that there is an added satisfaction in being able to share that part of the recovery process with their patients. Included with that is the opportunity to see fairly dramatic results if the patients come for help before their problems get too far along.

Podiatrists also report that they tend to have more autonomy than other medical professionals, that is to say, fewer people looking over their shoulders and second-guessing them. That independence is tied in with the ability to control their schedules in a way that other medical professionals sometimes envy. For the person seeking a good balance between work and personal life, podiatry is generally viewed as a great choice.

Another factor that looms large for many podiatrists is that the schooling and the required training that comes after, though extensive, takes less time than for other medical specialists. They also note that it tends to be more focused even in the first years of studies, in which class work is not very different from that of other medical disciplines.

In addition, podiatry school is less expensive to attend than other medical schools, a factor of great importance to many who grew up wanting to be doctors, but in families of only modest means. Podiatrists come out of school with less debt than many other medical professionals.

Podiatrists who practice surgery report that there is a good balance between the time they spend actually doing operations and the time they are in clinical mode. While surgeons tend to have strong feelings about the work they do, other podiatrists seem equally happy in meeting with patients, assessing and diagnosing their problems, and then treating them with methods other than surgery.

Podiatrists also tend to make excellent salaries and have the flexibility to live in a wide variety of environments. Salaries depend somewhat on location, and there are places where the concentration of podiatrists is quite high. There are far more places that are in significant need of podiatrists, where patients are willing to pay well for their services.

UNATTRACTIVE FEATURES

MANY PODIATRISTS SHARE THE COMPLAINT that their profession is not respected by other medical practitioners, despite their having to go through an extensive medical education and training process. Some podiatrists point directly at orthopedic physicians, saying that some in that specialty dislike podiatrists because they are both engaged in dealing with foot and ankle illnesses and injuries and are, in a sense, in competition.

There may be some truth to this. For example, the American Association of Orthopaedic Surgeons (AAOS) wrote to Congress opposing a bill that would have put podiatrists on the same pay scale as other doctors working in veterans' hospitals. The AAOS said that podiatrists have much less training and less experience than do orthopedic surgeons and should not be put in the same class with them.

There is also a tremendous sense of frustration that there is not enough emphasis on the part of the medical establishment on preventive care and for a more holistic approach to patient needs. So much unnecessary pain could be avoided if patients and the public in general could receive more encouragement to pay attention to their health maintenance before something goes wrong.

Another complaint, common in the health profession, is that there is too much paperwork, mostly related to insurance forms, to deal with. Also related to the business side of the profession are complaints about the medical supply companies. These include more annoying paperwork, as well as feeling pressured by the companies to try tools and procedures that are new and pricey.

Impatient patients are another of the challenges faced by podiatrists. From assessment, to treatment, to the end of the recovery period from injuries and illnesses of the feet and ankles can be a lengthy period of time. Podiatrists sometimes find themselves in a struggle with patients over taking the full recovery period. Too many try to get back on their feet too soon. Some podiatrists say that preventing relapses is one of the hardest jobs they have.

Physical exhaustion is another hazard of the job, especially for podiatrists who are also surgeons. Even if patients are cooperative, there is still handling of lower limbs that can be taxing. Many podiatrists would like to have more support staff available.

EDUCATION AND TRAINING

IN ORDER TO BECOME A PODIATRIST, one must have a Doctor of Podiatric Medicine (DPM) degree from an accredited college of podiatric medicine. The typical DPM degree program takes four years to complete, after you graduate from college.

It is typical for the prospective DPM student to already have a bachelor's degree with a science major. The undergraduate courses that a DPM school might require for admissions can include (with laboratory experience as part of each course):

Anatomy
Biochemistry
Biology

Cell Biology
Embryology
Evolution
General Chemistry
Genetics
Histology
Inorganic Chemistry
Microbiology
Organic Chemistry
Physics
Physiology
Zoology

In addition, admission to DPM programs requires a successful completion of the Medical College Admission Test (MCAT), strong grades, recommendations, and personal interviews.

There are only nine colleges that train students to be podiatrists. These schools are accredited by the Council on Podiatric Medical Education (CPME) and are permitted to officially be called a Podiatric Medical School. The nine podiatric schools are:

- Barry University School of Podiatric Medicine

- Arizona School of Podiatric Medicine at Midwestern University

- Des Moines University College of Podiatric Medicine and Surgery

- California School of Podiatric Medicine at Samuel Merritt University

- New York College of Podiatric Medicine

- Kent State University College of Podiatric Medicine, in Ohio

- Dr. William M. Scholl College of Podiatric Medicine, in Illinois, at Rosalind Franklin University

- Temple University School of Podiatric Medicine

- College of Podiatric Medicine, in California, at Western University of Health Sciences

There is one podiatric medical school in Canada, Université du Québec B Trois-RiviPres that offers the DPM degree. Its curriculum is based on the standards established by the CPME, although it has not been accredited by that US organization. However, the program has been accredited by the

Quebec Order of Podiatrists and L'Office des professions du Québec.

Students in a DPM program take courses similar to those taken by other medical students. Some of their specific courses include:

Biochemistry
Casting
Clinical Foot Orthopedics
Clinical Neurology
Community Health
Foot and Ankle Radiology
Fundamental Dermatology
Fundamentals of Practice
General Anatomy
General Orthopedics
Gerontology
Histology
Infectious Disease
Introduction to Surgery
Internal Medicine
Lower Extremity Anatomy
Medical Microbiology
Neurophysiology
Pathomechanics
Pediatric Orthopedics
Perioperative Protocol
Pharmacology
Physical Medicine
Physiology
Podiatric Surgical Skills
Principles of Digital and Metatarsal Surgery
Principles of First Ray Surgery
Principles of Pathology
Principles of Reconstructive Surgery of the Foot and Leg
Professional Administration and Development
Sports Medicine
The Law and Podiatric Medicine
Traumatology
Vascular Disease

In addition to their classroom courses, third and fourth year students add clinical rotations to their class work. The rotation process takes the students through different hospital departments so that they can experience a variety of medical specialties and – under the supervision of specialist physicians – treat patients with a broad spectrum of ailments. Students conduct physical examinations, update patient records, and even get to assist the doctors in performing surgeries and other procedures. As students in a podiatric program, you would see some extra time spent in clinics related to that profession. Rotations might take a student through such areas as:

- Anesthesia
- Diagnosis Clinic
- Orthopedic Clinic
- Podiatric Medicine
- Radiology
- Surgery Clinic
- Wound Care/Physical Medicine

Residency

After earning a DPM, podiatrists must apply to and complete a three-year podiatric medical and surgical residency (PMSR) program in order to complete their formal education. A residency takes place in a hospital and allows the new doctor to gain true hands-on experience and also begin to specialize in a focused component area of podiatry, such as sports medicine or gerontology. During your residency you will work under the supervision of an attending physician.

There are fewer than 250 residency programs in the US at this time. It is anticipated that there will be an expansion of the number of residencies accompanied by an increase in the number of DPM graduates being accepted into residencies so they can complete their training and become certified.

Licensing and Certification

Podiatrists in every state must be licensed, which requires passing the American Podiatric Medical Licensing Exam (APMLE). The exam, created by the National Board of Podiatric Medical Examiners, is accepted in all states, although several states require the DPM to pass a state-specific exam. In Canada, there are provincial licensing exams for podiatrists, as well as a national exam to become a licensed physician.

Although there is no requirement that they must, many podiatrists in the

US and Canada elect to become board certified, which is a way of expressing their commitment to the profession by undergoing rigorous testing of their knowledge in a series of written and oral exams. This is a voluntary process, but those who choose to do it feel that they are also saying to their patients that they are deeply committed and extremely knowledgeable. The certification process also requires a level of work experience as well as the exams.

There are three certifying boards in the US: the American Board of Foot and Ankle Surgery, the American Board of Podiatric Medicine, and the American Board of Multiple Specialties in Podiatry.

EARNINGS

THE MEDIAN ANNUAL EARNINGS FOR PODIATRISTS are about $120,000. That means half of these doctors earn more and half earn less. The lowest 10 percent of working podiatrists earn about $50,000, while the top percent earn more than $185,000.

Podiatrists are at the high end of the scale among all health diagnosing and treating practitioners who, as a whole, have a median salary of about $85,000.

Much of the potential earnings for a podiatrist depends on location. The swings from one state to another and even among the metropolitan areas within any one state can be considerable, often in tens of thousands of dollars. In the five states with the highest levels of employment for podiatrists – California, Florida, New York, Ohio, and Texas – the annual mean salary ranges from $115,000 in California to almost $170,000 in Texas.

The metropolitan areas that offer the highest annual salaries to podiatrists are Honolulu at $280,000; the Silver Spring-Frederick-Rockville, Maryland area at $260,000; St. Louis at $196,000; San Antonio at $190,000; and Milwaukee at about $185,000.

Salaries tend to be lower in those areas that have the highest location quotients, that is to say the highest concentrations of podiatrists as compared to the national average. For example, the Ft. Lauderdale area of Florida has a location quotient of 3.45, nearly three and a half times the number of podiatrists per population than average. The annual mean salary there is $132,000. For Warren-Troy-Farmington Hills, Michigan, which has the third highest location quotient for podiatrists at 2.59, the annual mean salary drops down to $100,000. The only metropolitan area with both a high location quotient (2.57) and an annual mean salary over $150,000 is Nassau County-Suffolk County, New York.

OUTLOOK

THERE ARE ABOUT 9,600 WORKING PODIATRISTS in the US. That is one for every 33,200 people in this country.

Podiatrists tend to be located in the more populated urban areas. Studies by the American Podiatric Medical Association and the Census Bureau found in recent years that in Florida and the Northeastern states the ratio of podiatrists to the total population ran as high as 45 per 100,000 while in the Southwest, Upper Midwest, and the Northern Plains states the ratios were more typically 16 per 100,000.

Looking down the road, the US population will continue to see a rising average age with a slower death rate, and the number of people who will have mobility and foot-related problems is expected to increase. More podiatrists will be needed to provide care for these older citizens as well as for that growing segment of the population with chronic conditions such as diabetes and obesity, both of which tend to limit the mobility of their sufferers and lead to the types of problems, such as poor circulation in the feet and lower extremities, that require podiatric care.

All data suggest that there should be a need for more persons to join this profession. Employment of podiatrists is projected to grow almost 15 percent in the coming decade, about double the average for all occupations. Nevertheless, as there are a relatively small number of people already in this profession, the fast growth rate will result in only about 1,400 new jobs in the US overall.

Opportunities will come from expanded openings in existing workplaces, a substantial part of that resulting from the retirement by the current generation of podiatrists. The number of podiatrists may increase more rapidly than predicted. At present, although there are only a few colleges training podiatrists, there are many graduates waiting for opportunities to work. The problem is a bottleneck for graduates with their DPM degrees because there are not enough openings in residency programs to accommodate them all. The individual DPM colleges and the American Podiatric Medical Association are working together to get more hospitals to offer residencies and are also working with current residency programs to expand the number of graduates they will accept.

GETTING STARTED

IF YOU CHOSE TO PURSUE A CAREER AS A PODIATRIST, you will find that you have a more limited number of options as far as the medical schools that offer the DPM degree. Once you do get into one of the nine schools, you will be on your way. However, as has already been noted, there is another and even more narrow bottleneck ahead – the limited number of residencies available to the students who graduate from the podiatric schools.

One of the most important things you can do, even as you prepare to go to a podiatric school for your degree, is to examine residencies where the school may have some affiliation. Most schools have connections with hospitals and clinics in their immediate area in which students make their initial contact with the realities of practicing podiatry while still pursuing their education in the classroom.

You can also review the websites of different schools to see the hospitals and clinics where they have affiliations. This can influence your choice of school. For example, you may be most interested in working with military veterans, so a school that has an affiliation with a veterans hospital would be your preference over one that does not. The same would hold true if you wanted to work with kids – you would want to find a school with an affiliation with a children's hospital.

The schools do not necessarily list all of the residencies in which their students have found places. However, some like the Barry University in Miami, Florida have a listing of all the places in which their graduates have found residencies. In the case of Barry students, the list is extensive and gives you an idea that the school is widely respected in all parts of the country and its graduates taken seriously. If a school does not have such a listing on its website, you can call and track the information down with school administrators.

You may also find that each of the schools offers special programs that are not a part of the standard curriculum but that may be of particular interest to you. Barry University's Podiatry School operates the Yucatan Crippled Children's Project in which its podiatrists, working alongside other healthcare professionals and public officials in Mexico bring medical care to the crippled children in the Yucatan as an ongoing project. The best fourth year students are occasionally invited to join the team. Barry also offers its students many opportunities to volunteer in other needy areas within the global community, which it sees as part of its institutional mission.

For more information on residencies, you can visit the website of the American Podiatric Medical Association. There are several sections on residencies, including how to prepare for an interview and related topics. You can even download the manual, *A Comprehensive Survival Guide to Securing a Residency*.

ORGANIZATIONS

■ **American Academy of Podiatric Sports Medicine**
www.aapsm.org

■ **American Association for Women Podiatrists**
www.aawpinc.com

■ **American Board of Multiple Specialties in Podiatry**
www.abmsp.org

■ **American College of Foot and Ankle Orthopedics and Medicine**
www.acfaom.org

■ **American College of Foot and Ankle Surgeons**
www.acfas.org

■ **American Podiatric Medical Association**
www.apma.org

■ **Canadian Federation of Podiatric Medicine**
www.podiatryinfocanada.ca

■ **Canadian Podiatric Medical Association**
www.podiatrycanada.org

■ **Council on Podiatric Medical Education**
www.cpme.org

■ Institute for Preventive Foot Health
www.ipfh.org

PUBLICATIONS

■ American Podiatry Magazine
http://americanpodiatrymagazine.com

■ Clinics in Podiatric Medicine and Surgery
www.podiatric.theclinics.com

■ Foot and Ankle Quarterly
www.datatrace.com/faq-27-annual-subscription.html

■ Journal of Bone and Joint Surgery
http://jbjs.org

■ Journal of Foot and Ankle Research
https://jfootankleres.biomedcentral.com

■ Journal of Foot and Ankle Surgery
www.jfas.org

■ Journal of the American Podiatric Medical Association
www.japmaonline.org

■ Podiatry Management Online
www.podiatrym.com

■ Podiatry Today
www.podiatrytoday.com

Copyright 2017 Institute For Career Research
Careers Internet Database Website www.careers-internet.org
Careers Reports on Amazon
www.amazon.com/Institute-For-Career-Research/e/B007DO4Y9E
For information please email service@careers-internet.org

www.ingramcontent.com/pod-product-compliance
Lightning Source LLC
Chambersburg PA
CBHW070720210526
45170CB00021B/1384